CRUSHING TYPE 1 AND 2 DIABETES WITH A VEGAN DIET

50 FOODS AND 14 FRUITS TO AID THE PROCESS OF RECOVERY

FRUITS AND FOOD ROUTINE FOR THE DIABECTICS

When you enter the doctor's office and you just hear the actual term, "diabetic diet" you might normally panic, however, you don't need to. There aren't any real diabetic diets available that you can be a part of. Nevertheless, a qualified dietary specialist as well as your physician can provide you with assistance and direction in the correct direction. This information will offer you a few tips and provide you with ideas to go over together with your physician and also the nutritional expert.

Once you have a while to adapt to the thought of being diabetic, contact your physician and obtain some good info regarding how to eat correctly to regulate the diabetes. Because there are absolutely no specific diet plans to make use of regarding diabetes you are able to develop one which can particularly meet your needs. The very first thing to consider is the fact that when you've got diabetes it's not necessary to give up consuming all you usually eat you need to simply try to eat them in a different way.

Several things you are able to change in your own eating routine is:

1. Just how much you consume

2. While you eat

3. The way you make your own meals

4. Lower sugar as well as treats

5. Look at exactly how as well as when you consume carbohydrate food

6. Increase the examples below:

• Fruits

- Vegetables

- Wholemeal wheat cereals

7. Minimize unwanted fat consumption

8. Moderation in alcohol consumption

When you're attempting to adapt to the diabetic diet Plan keep an eye on just how much you typically consume at mealtime

and when you might have snack foods during the day. If you do not consume frequent meals, in that case it's essential for you to create a diet program. You will need to see to it that you're consuming breakfast every day, lunch time meal, and evening meal together with smaller snack food items between main meal times. It's important to keep to a minimum of 1600 calorie diet every single day. If you're accustomed to consuming a substantial amount of food then you'll have to scale back slightly at each and every meal. Incorporating smaller snack food items throughout the day may help fill the particular emptiness within your stomach.

This can accomplish beneficial things for you personally. It helps maintain your sugar level. Help keep your cravings in check. As well as prevent you from pigging out whenever you sit down to enjoy a regular planned meal.

A very advantageous and beneficial thing regarding eating such as this, together with physical exercise, it helps you to definitely reduce weight. It will not only assist in the short-term, but when you get accustomed to this, you will discover you will keep the extra weight off. In addition you might very well observe a general boost in your own personal overall health.

You should definitely consume breakfast each and every morning and then try to incorporate a bit of fresh fruit. Fruit flesh not just tastes great, but it's perfect for providing you with vigor and it will be a terrific snack. It's important too, that you diligently consume lunch every single day to assist you uphold a comfortable quantity of energy all through your entire day regardless of what you're up to. If you're a person who typically cuts out lunch consider beginning by simply having a few crackers or perhaps a salad for lunch break so that you will eat some thing and it'll become a light snack.

Your next crucial meal you should take in will be dinner. Whenever you eat dinner attempt to consume a well-balanced meal so your entire body is not going to feel really over stuffed or heavy. It's also vital that you get your meals at standard arranged times every single day so your body may adjust and also process your food before going to bed. Take care not to eat very early. By eating ahead of time in the actual evening you might end up famished once again and wish to eat prior to going to bed. There's just one final suggestion to offer on regarding your own diabetic meals. Which is exactly how you cook your own foods. You need to broil or even bake the lean meats. Additionally if you need to cook food on top of the actual range make use of Virgin Organic Olive Oil instead of butter and various other Tran's fat packed food items. As you have seen any diabetic diet program is definitely not the actual end of the world. Actually if it's observed, you'll hold off the actual deterioration of the diabetes, shed weight and also enhance your all around health general

Diabetes is no fun; it can make you unwell, increase the risk of many other conditions and reduce your quality of life. The good news is, type 2 diabetes is preventable and, should you happen to have it already, potentially reversible.

Diet is the key. More and more health professionals now recommend a substantial diet change and many type 2 diabetic patients are successfully reversing their condition.

The big issue in diabetes is high blood sugar, a result of the body's sugar metabolism – governed by the hormone insulin – working incorrectly. This has a knock-on effect on other systems in the body, increasing blood cholesterol and fat levels, damaging the eyes, kidneys and nerve endings and can lead to insensitivity in hands and feet.

Type 2 diabetes is usually (but not always) linked to increased body weight and especially to abdominal obesity. When the body's metabolism can't keep up with the amount and type of food eaten, droplets of fat are stored under the skin, but also in muscle and liver cells. Where and how you store fat is largely genetic. When the amount of fat in the cells reaches a certain level, it reduces the cells' ability to react to insulin correctly, leading to insulin resistance. Studies show the resistance in muscles and the liver is strongly linked to fat storage in these tissues.

With the right kind of diet, you can not only prevent this happening, but also treat the condition. Studies where type 2 diabetics were prescribed a combination of diet change and mild exercise resulted in them being able to discontinue or significantly reduce medicating, in as little as three weeks!

The research is convincing – a wholesome, low-fat vegan diet is the best for reversing type 2 diabetes. It helps the body reduce fat stores in its cells, improves blood sugar control, reduces blood cholesterol, helps to induce weight loss without restricting portion sizes, prevents continued kidney and nerve damage and helps to lower blood pressure.

The usefulness of vegan diets was even endorsed by the American Diabetes Association in their 2010 Clinical Practice Guidelines.

Basic principles of the diet

1st principle – no animal products

By eliminating all animal products you avoid eating substantial amounts of fat and your cholesterol intake will be zero. Most of the fat found in animal products is saturated and there's absolutely no requirement for saturated fat in our diet.

Another good reason for avoiding all animal products is because animal protein from meat, fish, dairy and eggs places an additional strain on the kidneys and can increase the damage already caused by diabetes. Protecting kidneys is a key issue for diabetics.

All foods should be of plant origin and unrefined wherever possible, which means they will be naturally high in fibre and complex carbohydrates. Animal products contain no fibre or healthy carbohydrates, while plant foods (supplemented with vitamin

B12) contain all the essential nutrients we need.

Second principle – low-fat

Even though plant fats are healthier, it is important to keep them to a minimum. In order to reverse or improve diabetes it is essential to reduce fat stores inside the cells and this can only happen if you avoid excessive fat consumption.

The amount of fat per serving should be three grams maximum (just 10 per cent of calories should come from fat). Apart from added oils, you might need to curb the amount of nuts and seeds you eat. Within the low-fat rule, the best sources of healthy, omega-3 fats are flaxseed, hempseed and walnuts (for snacking or adding to dishes) and rapeseed oil for cooking.

Third principle – low glycemic index (GI)

Glycemic index (GI) is a measure of how carbohydrates in food affect your blood sugar. Carbohydrates that are digested fast and rapidly release glucose into the blood and have a high GI. Carbohydrates that break down slowly, releasing glucose gradually into the bloodstream, have a low GI.

To help the body use energy effectively and prevent sugar highs and lows, it's important to focus on slow-releasing, low-GI foods. But bear in mind that it's the overall GI that counts, so you can combine low and medium GI foods to achieve the desired lower GI effect.

Low GI foods include: most fruits and vegetables, pulses (beans, soya, peas, lentils, chickpeas), barley, buckwheat, hummus, pasta, nuts and seeds, sweet potatoes, dried apricots and prunes, rolled oats, all-bran cereals, wholegrain pumpernickel bread, soya yoghurt.

Medium GI foods include: wholemeal and rye bread, crispbread, brown rice, basmati rice, corn, porridge oats, shredded wheat, pineapple, cantaloupe melon, figs, raisins and beans in tomato sauce.

High GI foods (to avoid) include: potatoes, rice cakes, watermelon, pumpkin, white bread, white rice, cornflakes, sweet cereal, dates and sugary foods.

A vegan diet based on these principles is the healthiest possible, but it is advised you take a vitamin B12 supplement or eat enough B12 enriched foods. Vitamin B12 requirements may be higher in diabetics taking the drug Metformin as it can reduce B12 absorption.

Whether you're at risk of or have type 2 diabetes, your diet should be based on wholegrains, pulses, soya, vegetables, fruit and nuts and seeds. This limits the types of food you can eat, but not the amount. Being high in fibre and digested gradually, it makes you feel full sooner and for longer and the calorie intake is reduced by the minimal amount of fat it contains. Research shows that diabetics who follow this type of vegan diet get better results than any single drug can produce!

50 Best Foods for Diabetics

For most of us, dialing back on sugar and simple carbs is an effective way to fast-track weight loss. But for those living with diabetes, it can be a matter of life and death. That's why it's important to know the best foods for diabetics (and which foods diabetics should be mindful of).

Diabetics are two to four times more likely than people without diabetes to die of heart disease or experience a life-threatening stroke, according to the American Heart Association. And for those who don't properly control their condition, the odds of health issues—which range from cardiovascular trouble to nerve damage and kidney disease—increases exponentially.

Luckily there are plenty of delicious foods that are compatible with diabetes.

The best foods for diabetics are low-carb, low-sugar, and high in fiber, digestion-slowing macronutrients like healthy fats and protein, and high in flavor. These diabetes foods are recommended by registered dietitians and certified diabetes educators:

1. Quinoa

This nutty, trendy whole grain is a good source of fiber and protein, making it a smart pick for a diabetes diet, Sarah Koszyk, RDN tells us. "With the fiber and protein combination found in quinoa, you'll feel fuller and have better blood sugar control. Protein also helps with the uptake of carbohydrates so the body can process them more easily. I suggest enjoying quinoa in a salad or casserole."

2. 100% Whole Wheat bread

Elizabeth Snyder, RD, LD, CDE says you can still eat carbs if you're diabetic. You just have to watch out for portion sizes: "The trouble [with eating carbs as a diabetic] lies in eating more carbohydrates than we need, as the body will choose to store any extra energy as fat," she says. So, rather of cutting out carbs entirely, Snyder recommends switching to complex carbs, such as 100% whole wheat bread, which are higher in vitamins, minerals, and blood-sugar-managing fiber than their simple, refined counterparts.

3. Beans

"Beans provide a notable combination of plant protein and soluble fiber that can help boost feelings of fullness and manage blood sugar levels," Jackie Newgent, RDN, culinary nutritionist, and author of The All-Natural Diabetes Cookbook explains. "Replacing some meat with beans can play a helpful role in heart health," which is particularly important for diabetics as heart disease is one of the most common complications of diabetes. Consider adding kidney beans to soups and black beans to your casseroles to boost your intake of the legumes.

4. Lentils

Lentils are rich in something called resistant starch: a type of carb that has a very minimal impact on your blood sugar levels because it passes through the body undigested and ultimately ends up feeding the healthy bacteria at the bottom of your digestive tract. So, not only will lentils help keep your blood sugar levels more even-keeled, they'll also help to improve your gut health.

5. Wild Salmon

"Salmon is a smart addition to anyone's eating plan, but for individuals with diabetes, it's especially beneficial," Lori Zanini, RD, CDE tells us. Here's why: "It's a healthy protein source that will not raise blood sugar levels and will help to decrease the risk of heart disease and stroke—a major concern for diabetics." Salmon's heart-healthy qualities come from its high levels of omega-3 fatty acids. This particular fat reduces levels of triglycerides, a risk factor for coronary heart disease, according to a review in the journal Endocrine Practice.

6. Greek Yogurt

Looking for a protein-packed way to fuel your morning? Greek yogurt is the answer. "It naturally contains both carbohydrates and protein, which is a perfect combination to help control hunger levels and blood sugars," says

Koszyk. "Plus, choosing Greek yogurt will give you more protein and fewer carbohydrates than regular yogurt, which can help better control blood-sugar levels. Enjoy yogurt in a smoothie or as a snack paired with some berries and chia seeds."

7. Spinach

"Leafy greens, like spinach, are great non-starchy vegetable options because they contain lutein, an important nutrient for eye health. This nutrient is essential for people with diabetes since they have a higher risk for blindness than those without diabetes," explains Newgent. That's not all spinach has going for it. A study published in the journal Archives of Internal Medicine found that adults who consumed 4,069 milligrams of potassium per day had a 37 percent lower risk of heart disease compared to those who consumed only 1,793 milligrams. Just one cup of cooked spinach contains 839 milligrams of potassium (which is equivalent to what's in 2 medium bananas) or 20 percent of that target intake.

8. Berries

Craving a treat? Consider berries your go-to when your sweet tooth strikes. "Strawberries, blueberries, raspberries, and blackberries are all low on the glycemic index and are considered to be superfoods for diabetics," Koszyk explains. The combination of being low in sugar and high in fiber contributes to their diabetes-friendly ability to gradually raise blood sugars. An added bonus: according to two recent animal studies, consuming a diet rich in polyphenols—a naturally occurring chemical found abundantly in berries—can decrease the formation of fat cells by up to 73 percent!

9. Broccoli

"Cruciferous vegetables like kale, broccoli, cauliflower, brussels sprouts and cabbage are high in something called sulforaphane," Miriam Jacobson, RD, CDN says. "The compound helps reduce oxidative stress and vascular complications associated with diabetes like heart disease and neuropathy, a term used to describe a problem with the nerves."

10.   Ground Flaxseeds

Add a satisfying crunch to your favorite oatmeal, salad, soup, or smoothie with the help of ground flaxseeds, a potent superfood for people with diabetes. "Ground flaxseeds contain lignans (a plant-based chemical compound) and fiber which help maintain blood sugar levels and glycemic control," Koszyk explains.

11.   Raw almonds

"I often recommend an ounce of almonds as a snack," Zanini tells us. "Almonds don't raise blood sugar levels and are a great source of magnesium, a nutrient that improves insulin sensitivity."

12.   Chia Seeds

"Chia seeds are a heart-healthy fat that contains fiber and omega-3s," Koszyk explains. "Research suggests that chia seeds help control blood glucose. And it's all thanks to the fiber content slowing the passage of glucose into the blood. Also, fiber fills us up which reduces our appetite and helps us eat less." Koszyk suggests enjoying chia seeds in yogurt, fruit and veggie smoothies, or salads.

13.   Avocado

What's better than avocado toast? Perhaps it's the fact that this fatty fruit can help you maintain healthy blood sugar levels, making it one of the best foods for diabetics watching their blood glucose levels. "Avocados contain a significant amount of healthful fats and dietary fiber, which help slow carbohydrate digestion and absorption and prevent spikes in blood sugar," Newgent tells us.

14.   Extra Virgin Olive Oil

It's time to upgrade your cooking oil. Extra virgin olive oil is rich in monounsaturated fats, which studies show can actually help lower levels of 'bad' LDL cholesterol. This is particularly important since diabetics have a higher risk of experiencing a heart attack or stroke. And get this: Snyder says losing just 7 percent of your body weight (if you're overweight) can result in significant health benefits for diabetics. Luckily for you, EVOO is rich in oleic acid, which a Journal of Lipid Research study found helps reduce lipogenesis, or fat formation.

15.   Peanut Butter

"When living with diabetes, eating a filling breakfast is an essential way to start the day," says Erin Spitzberg, MS, RDN, CDE, and author of Eat Like a Normal Person. "Adding a little fat for added satiety can help," she explains. She recommends pairing up your favorite breakfast carb—either a slice of whole grain toast, bowl of steel-cut oats, or high-fiber cereal—with 1 tablespoon of natural peanut butter. "The peanut butter adds approximately five grams of fat, which will help slow digestion and keep you full a little longer."

16.   Kale

Kale is called a superfood for good reason! Rich in fiber—with 16 grams, or over 60 percent of your daily recommended intake, of the digestion-slowing nutrient in just one cup—and low on the glycemic index, kale can help improve blood glucose control.

17.   Garlic

Despite what you may think, nixing sugar or salt doesn't have to be synonymous with bland, cardboard-like dishes. "So often, we think about what we can't eat when we start cutting out sugar. Instead, focus on ways to add more flavor to the foods you are eating," suggests Zanini. "There are so many great ways to add flavor without adding sugar or salt." Add a couple of crushed cloves of garlic to your marinara sauce or saute broccoli in a blend of extra virgin olive oil, chopped garlic, and crushed red pepper flakes.

18.   Cinnamon

A series of reviews printed in the American Journal of Clinical Nutrition discovered that adding a heaping teaspoon of cinnamon to a starchy meal like overnight oats could help stabilize blood sugar, ward off insulin spikes, and decrease fasting blood sugar. Experts believe that the spice's powerful antioxidants, known as polyphenols, are at work; these active compounds have been proven to improve insulin sensitivity and, in turn, your body's ability to store fat and manage hunger cues.

19.   Tuna Fish

Want to continue munching on your favorite crackers without fretting too much over your blood sugar levels? Consider pairing the crunchy snack with a can of tuna. Depending on the amount of healthy fats and protein you pair with your carb-laden snack, your body can digest the carbs much slower than you could if you ate the carbs alone. In fact, Tufts University researchers recently presented the results of a study which found that eating protein- and fat-rich tuna fish with a slice of white bread produced a slower rise in blood sugar than when eating carbs alone.

20.   Asparagus

Your favorite grilled veggie is more than just a tasty side. Because asparagus is rich in folate—just four spears contain 89 micrograms of the nutrient, or roughly 22 percent of your recommended daily value—it's one of the best foods for diabetics. According to a meta-analysis published in Diabetes Research and Clinical Practice, folic acid supplementation can lower cardiovascular risk among patients with Type 2 diabetes by reducing homocysteine levels, an amino acid that's been linked to increased risk of mortality when present in high levels in diabetic patients.

21.   Red Onion

Trust us: it's worth the tears. A Canadian study published in the American Journal of Clinical Nutrition discovered that a type of gut-healthy insoluble fiber found in onions, called oligofructose, can increase levels of ghrelin—a hormone that controls hunger—and lower levels of blood sugar. This allium can help diabetics in another way, as well. Thanks to their bioactive sulfur-containing compounds, onions can help lower cholesterol, ward off hardening of the arteries, and help maintain healthy blood pressure levels, according to a study published in the Evidence-Based Complementary and Alternative Medicine.

Pro tip: Eat your onions raw whenever you can for better benefits; a Journal of Agricultural and Food Chemistry study found the cholesterol-lowering properties were stronger in onions that were raw compared to those eaten cooked. Think: pico de gallo, sliced onions on sandwiches and burgers, or served in a Greek cucumber and tomato salad.

22.   Zucchini

If you love spaghetti and meatballs, swapping in veggies for grains should be your go-to move if you have diabetes. "Zucchini noodles and spaghetti squash are both easy and delicious ways to lower the amount of carbohydrates in some of your favorite dishes," says Zanini.

23.   Green Tea

Zanini is a huge fan of green tea—and with good reason. Because it is hydrating and filling, green tea can help prevent overeating, which will both stabilize blood sugar levels and aid weight loss efforts by boosting feelings of satiety. "This drink also increases your metabolism and reduces fat storage," Zanini adds.

24.   Oats

"Oats contain a type of fiber called beta-glucan, which seems to have an anti-diabetic effect," explains Newgent. Specifically, a review published in Vascular Health and Risk Management concluded that beta-glucans help to reduce high blood sugar and blood pressure, adding, "I advise people with diabetes to steer clear of added sugars by enjoying savory rather than sweet oatmeal." Try making oatmeal overnight with one of our overnight oats recipes for weight loss.

25.   Cauliflower

Check out the power of the cauliflower. Grate it up, and cauliflower rice is a great low-carb substitute for refined white rice, which can help keep your blood sugar levels more stable. Plus, cauliflower is rich in sulforaphane: a compound which a Science

Translational Medicine study found can inhibit glucose production in cells and improves glucose tolerance in rodents on high-fat or high-fructose diet.

26.   Broccoli Sprouts

You may not think much of broccoli sprouts when they pop up on your salad or sandwich, but these little guys are a powerful anti-inflammatory. They're packed with sulforaphane, which may help protect against cancer according to a study published in Cancer Prevention Research. Rich in fiber, broccoli sprouts are "a potent detoxifier and play a role in decreasing cancer risk," says Nicole Anziani, MS, RD, CDN, CDE and Clinical Manager at Fit4D.

27.   Edamame

"Edamame delivers a unique nutrition profile that could offer multiple benefits for those living with diabetes," Jenna Braddock, RDN, CSSD, sports dietitian and blogger at MakeHealthyEasy. "First, the fiber content of one cup is a staggering 10 grams, which could be very helpful in regulating blood sugar spikes and also contributes to reducing risk for heart disease. Second, as a plant-based source of protein, it could help reduce disease risk factors when it replaces meat in the diet. Lastly, edamame is a good source of the essential nutrient choline, and research shows that 9 out of ten Americans don't get enough of in the diet. Choline is important for helping to reduce homocysteine levels in the blood, a marker connected to increased risk of heart disease and connected to vascular disease in diabetes."

28.   Carrots

Instead of reaching for pretzels, chips, or another high-carb, high-calorie snack, carrots make for a healthy, low-calorie alternative. They are packed with vitamins C, D, E, and K, and the antioxidant beta-carotene, and make for a good low-carb snack when dunked in hummus or guacamole.

29.   Eggs

Eggs are a great source of protein. Anziani recommends opting for pasture-raised, organic omega-3 eggs. "The yolk will concentrate the omega-

3 fed to the chickens," she says, adding that these eggs are "a good source of choline and protein, but limit to under five per week."

30.   Tomatoes

Instead of choosing starchier veggies that can raise blood sugar, Anziani likes tomatoes to add to a salad or as a snack for a flavorful option that's low-calorie. They are also a good source of the antioxidant lycopene, which can help fight inflammation.

31.   Sardines

These fatty fish are some of the healthiest cold water fish, says Anziani. "[Sardines are] extremely convenient to eat when packaged as boneless and skinless in extra virgin olive oil," she says. Pour them over a salad with the olive oil dressing for a boost of healthy fats and protein to keep your blood sugar stable.

32.   Hummus

Instead of fattier cheese or mayo, Anziani recommends hummus as a dip for veggies or low-carb crackers.

"[Hummus] contains protein and a lot of taste for lower glycemic snacking," she says.

33.   Organic Tofu & Tempeh

Although vegetarians might have a tougher time getting protein in their diet, Anziani recommends organic tofu. Tofus absorbs the flavor of whatever it is cooked with, making it extremely versatile. Another high-protein option is tempeh, a fermented soy protein that can replace animal protein. However, those with a thyroid condition should only consume tofu or tempeh two to three times a week.

34.   Sweet Potato

Anziani says that although sweet potatoes are starchy, they're rich in beta-carotene, which is converted into the essential vitamin A. Sweet potatoes are also lower on the glycemic index than regular white potatoes, cementing their place among the best foods for diabetics. Treat sweet potatoes as your main starch for the meal and stick to a serving size—about ½ a cup baked or roasted. Keep the skin on for extra fiber.

35.   MCT Oil

MCT oil, named for the medium-chain triglycerides, a type of fatty acids, has been praised for its brain-boosting benefits, but it can also be used in small amounts to replace other fat sources. "MCT oil can be used in smoothies or drizzled over salads," Anziani says, "It is tasteless and may be used as fuel preferentially, versus being stored as fat."

36.	Pumpkin

Stock up on fresh pumpkin and pumpkin puree during the fall season. This super squash is rich in beta-carotene and adds a boost of seasonal flavor. "It can be a nice addition to oatmeal, yogurt, smoothies, or cooked as the starch component of dinner," Anziani says.

37.	Dark Chocolate

Watching your blood sugar doesn't mean you have to give up dessert entirely. Dark chocolate that's 70% cacao or above can have health benefits without spiking blood sugar; just pay attention to the ingredients and nutrition label. "One ounce or square can be consumed per day to strategically lower the stress hormone cortisol and keep milk chocolate cravings at bay," Anziani, says. Cacao is also rich in antioxidants, which can help fight inflammation.

38.   Shirataki Noodles

Even diabetics can enjoy pasta. Shirataki noodles are made from yam flour for a low-carb and super low-calorie option. "These noodles have 0-

20 calories per package and can be prepared in meals that would call for carby noodles," Anziani says.

39.   Bok Choy

"All vegetables are good sources of nutrition but dark green leafy vegetables like kale, spinach, bok choy, mustard, and broccoli provide vitamins like A, C, E, K and folate as well as fiber, iron and several minerals like calcium," Byron Richard, MS, RD, CDE, Clinical Nutrition Manager UC San Diego Health, says, "Leafy greens, as most non-starchy vegetables, have a low GI are low in calories and carbohydrates."

40.   Celery

Celery is an alkaline food that makes for an easy snack; Anziani likes that celery is nearly calorie-free. Slice up some celery to dip in hummus or fill with almond or peanut butter.

41.   Vegan Protein Powder

Smoothies, especially those with a lot of fruit, can have too much sugar for diabetics. But a good high-quality, low-sugar vegan protein powder can be an excellent meal replacement when shaken with unsweetened almond or coconut milk says Anziani. We like Vega One All-In-One Nutritional Shake Blend ($51.99 for large tun on Amazon). Each scoop is 137 calories, 11 grams of carbs, 2 grams of sugar, 6 grams of fiber and 15 grams of protein. Blend a low-sugar, high-protein smoothie with spinach, chia seeds, unsweetened almond milk, and a handful of berries for sweetness.

42.   Bitter Melon

Bitter melons aren't all that common; after all, as the name suggests, they are very bitter, Anziani says. However, she adds that it has been proven to lower blood sugar. A study published in the Journal of Ethnopharmacology found that 2,000 milligrams of bitter melon a day lowers blood glucose levels in people with type 2 diabetes.

43.   Seltzer

Instead of sodas and sweetened beverages, which can pack up to 40 grams of sugar per serving and can wreak havoc on blood sugar levels, Anziani recommends opting for unsweetened seltzer instead. Try a low-calorie flavored brand like Spindrift, or buy plain club soda or seltzer and flavor yourself with a squeeze of lemon, lime, or fresh mint sprigs.

44.   Walnuts

Nuts are some of the best foods for diabetics since they are low in carbs, high in healthy fats, and high in fiber. Walnuts are one of the best nuts available because of their high omega-

3 content Anziani says—one serving (about ¼ a cup) has almost 3 grams of omega-3s. Just be sure to stick to one serving size so as not to go overboard on calories.

45.   Chickpeas

Like other beans, chickpeas are a high-fiber legume that can be eaten instead of animal protein, Anziani recommends. Roasted and seasoned chickpeas also make for a good high-fiber, low-carb snack compared to other high glycemic options such as pretzels and potato chips.

46.	Flax Crackers

Instead of other high-carb crackers, opt for high-fiber flax crackers. They're an excellent base for hummus, guacamole, or turkey slices. We like Mary's Gone Crackers Super Seed Crackers which are just 160 calories per serving and have 19 grams of carbs, 3 grams of fiber, 0 grams of sugar, and 3 grams of protein.

47.	Bone Broth

Bone broth is rich in collagen, which can make for a protein-packed and satiating snack and one of the best foods for diabetics, Anziani says. Sip some warm broth for an afternoon snack to keep you satisfied until dinnertime. We like Pacific Foods for a tasty and affordable option.

48.   Lean Chicken

Combining proteins are key in keeping your blood sugar down while also leaving you feeling satisfied. Anziani recommends a lean protein like chicken because it's nearly pure protein, highly satiating, and versatile for a variety of recipes. "A good portion of protein is a palm-sized piece at meals, or about 22 grams per meal," she says.

49.   Wild Rice

You don't have to give up rice entirely if you're diabetic. Anziani likes wild rice because it's high in fiber. She says it's an ancient grain that is actually a grass and is high in manganese, zinc, iron, and folate.

50.   Bell Peppers

Red, green, orange, and yellow bell peppers aren't just colorful additions to your salad; they can be a blood sugar-friendly snack all on their own.

They have a sweeter taste without the sugar content of most fruit (about 3 grams of sugar per medium bell pepper). Anziani also likes how they are rich in vitamin C and also have a satisfying crunch. Slice them up and enjoy them as a snack with hummus or guacamole.

FRUITS FOR DIABECTICS

The 14 best fruits for type 1 and type 2 diabetes

The fruits listed below are your dietary MVPs. You'll want to celebrate their greatness by hoisting them in the air... or just by eating them regularly. All of them have a GI of 55 or below and a GL under 10 per serving.

1. Apples

Apples provide healthy fiber, which is important for, you know, staying regular. They're tasty on their own or with a tablespoon of all-natural peanut butter.

2. Bananas

Bananas are an inexpensive and delicious way to get some potassium and vitamin C.

Be sure to eat your bananas as soon as they're ripe (or even while they're still a little green). The longer they sit and the browner they get, the sweeter they become. True story — according to a 1992 study, this raises the sugar content and the GI.

Remember that half a medium banana is the recommended serving size.

3. Pears

Pre-PEAR yourself! Pears are loaded with antioxidants, vitamins, and minerals. And red-skinned pears contain carotenoids, which are thought to reduce the risk of certain cancers and eye disease. What's not to love?

4. Prunes (pitted)

In addition to possibly being your grandma's favorite fruit, prunes are one of the lowest-GI fruits. Plus, they're a natural remedy for constipation and are rich in antioxidants. Generally, two to three prunes is considered a serving.

5. Strawberries

Sweet, sweet berries are actually very low on the GI index. Eating 1 cup of strawberries can also protect your heart, increase your HDL (good) cholesterol level, and decrease your LDL (bad) cholesterol level.

Limit these medium-GI fruits

These fruits are OK to eat in smaller portions. Reach for them less often than the low-GI fruits listed above. They have a GI of 56 to 69 and a GL under 11.

6. Apricots

Fresh apricots might not be your usual go-to fruit, but they have a certain zing you can't get anywhere else. Enjoy them on their own or try grilling them and eating them with a protein like chicken.

7. Grapes

One cup of grapes is a healthy way to get some fiber, vitamin C, and vitamin K. They're also easy to enjoy right out of the bag (just wash them first!) and a great addition to your packed lunch.

8. Kiwi

Kiwi is an excellent source of vitamins E and K, folate, and potassium. Try slicing up a small kiwi to enjoy with some protein-rich Greek yogurt for breakfast.

Time-saving tip: You don't need to peel kiwis to eat them. Their skin is edible. Just make sure to wash them before you dig in.

9. Pineapple

Pineapple is a delicious source of bromelain (an anti-inflammatory), and it's also rich in vitamin C. Try pairing it with a protein like cottage cheese.

10. Blueberries:

Blueberries get their deep pigment from anthocyanins, a type of flavonoid, known particularly to lower the risk of diabetes.

11. Guava:

It's a great snack for diabetics with a low glycemic index. Guava is very rich in dietary fiber that helps ease constipation (a common diabetic complaint) and can lower the chance of developing type-2 diabetes.

12. Watermelon:

The high potassium content makes watermelon one of best fruits for proper kidney functioning which in turn keep your blood uric acid levels on the lower side. This prevents kidney damage especially if you are diabetic.

Also, diabetes can cause nerve damage but lycopene found in watermelon really helps reduce the effect.

13. Papaya

Natural antioxidants within the fruit make papaya a great choice for diabetics. Diabetics are prone to many ailments, including heart or nerve damage caused by irregular blood sugar levels. A diet incorporating papaya can obstruct future cell damage for a better and longer life span.

14. Oranges:

The flavonols, flavanones and phenolic acid found in oranges, have shown tremendous protective abilities, and especially in diabetics. When it comes to glucose metabolism, citrus fruits not only slow glucose update, but also inhibit the movement or transport of glucose through the intestines and liver.

Being a diabetic should never stop you from eating fruits. The key is to eat a wide variety to keep your body toxin-free benefiting from their important role in detoxification. There is no need for exotic fruits, eating fruits that are fresh, local and in season are best suited for you.